THE SMILOGIE METHOD

"Even in the hardest times, your smile matters."

A GENTLE DEDICATION

For my sisters
whose love has been a quiet anchor.

For every woman walking this path
may these pages serve as a companion
—and a reminder that you are not alone.

*“Thank you for being here —
and for trusting these pages
to walk beside you.”*

Published by Smilogie trading as IDWO Ltd.

Edited by Pauline Pascarelli

This guide is intended for supportive and informational purposes only. It is not a substitute for professional medical advice, diagnosis, or treatment. Always seek the advice of your doctor, oncology team, or another qualified healthcare provider with any questions you have regarding a medical condition or treatment.

Smilogie and The Smilogie Method are original works created by Isabelle (Isy) de Wouters d'Oplinter.

Cover and content design @BeaReisCustodio

Printed via Amazon KDP First edition, 2026

ISBN 978-1-0682496-3-1 (paperback)
ISBN 978-1-0682496-4-8 (hardback)
ISBN 978-1-0682496-5-5 (ebook)

www.thesmilogiemethod.co

@thesmilogiemethod

Contents

Safety Note

This guide is for education and reflection. It is not a substitute for medical advice, diagnosis, or treatment. Always discuss treatments, medications, and supplements with your oncology or menopause team.

Clinicians and educators are welcome to share brief, unmodified excerpts for patient education, provided clear attribution is given to *The Smilogie Method*.

"One smile today.

One moment of ease.

One step forward."

Welcome

If you are reading this, life has likely handed you something you never asked for — a diagnosis, a shift, a sudden new chapter. Before anything else, I want you to know: you are not alone.

This book was born from real conversations — in waiting rooms, on long nights, in quiet kitchens. It gathers everything I wished existed when life wobbled: clarity, comfort, and the courage to keep smiling.

Cancer has touched too many — from my grandparents to my mother, to the women I have walked besides as a coach. I've seen the fear, the fatigue, the strength and the quiet courage it brings out of us.

I have also navigated my own wobbles and anxiety through perimenopause, wondering if I would ever feel steady, "me" again.

Life has a way of testing us —twists and turns and those relentless *"what now?"* moments. In the middle of my own struggles, I remembered a saying which carried me through some of the darkest of times:

"Smile, and the world smiles with you.
Cry, and it cries with you."

It was not about **pretending** everything was fine. It was about **allowing** myself just one little smile — soft, quiet and at times even shaky. Each time something shifted, and a little strength returned.

I wanted something that met women where they are — tired, brave, sometimes anxious, always human.

That is how the Smilogie Method was born. Not from theory, but from real moments. Mine, my family's, and the women I have been honoured to support.

It is about micro-practices that calm the body, ease the mind, and gently remind the heart of its strength.

Smilogie is not about faking positivity.

It is about finding safety in small things: a breath, a pause, a smile which belongs only to you.

This little guide is here as a small companion to sit with you in waiting rooms, to ease long nights, and to remind you that healing is not only about treatment, but about kindness toward yourself.

Inside, you'll find:

- Gentle explanations of how cancer treatment and hormones intertwine
- Ways to ease body, mind, and heart wobbles
- Smilogie tools for rest, energy, intimacy, and emotional calm
- Tiny practices and affirmations to bring you back to yourself

These practices are grounded in mindfulness, lifestyle medicine, and psycho-oncology research — yet written in plain, gentle language.

This guide is not about doing everything. It is about what feels right *today*.

Even one small smile can be enough to begin the shift.
And by holding this book, you have already started.

Your courage brought you here. Let this little book remind you to rest, to smile, and to begin again — softly.

Isy x

How to Use This Little Guide

No rules.

Let this book sit quietly beside you.

- Read straight through when you want a gentle companion
- Bring it to appointments and use a tab to anchor questions
- Open anywhere on days that feel wobbly

Linger where something lands—an affirmation, a note, a line that lets you breathe easier.

Take what helps; leave the rest.

This is your companion.

What You will Find Inside

Every tab offers something a little different. Some bring practical tools and insights; others invite you to pause, breathe, and reflect. Many hold a blend of both—pages that bring clarity and pages that bring comfort. Each one is here for you, designed with your well-being and strength in mind.

1. A GENTLE REFRESHER

Understanding how breast and gynaecological cancers shift your hormones.

2. TREATMENT & HORMONES

Making sense of surgery, chemotherapy, radiotherapy, and hormone therapies.

3. DOCTOR VISITS

Questions, notes and trackers to help you feel clear and confident at appointments.

4. BODY WOBBLES

Hot flushes, dryness, fatigue, bone, skin and digestion changes.

5. MIND WOBBLES

Anxiety, scan anxiety, brain fog and identity shifts.

6. HEART WOBBLES

Relationships, intimacy, fertility, grief and tenderness.

7. NURTURE & NUTRITION

Gentle guidance on food, hydration, supplements and small rituals.

8. ENERGY & REST

Pacing, sleep and restorative practices when energy is scarce.

9. REDISCOVERY BEYOND TREATMENT

Rebuilding joy, identity and confidence — step by step.

10. REFLECTIONS & SMILOGIE TOUCHSTONES

Journaling prompts and gentle reminders to reconnect with yourself.

11. USEFUL RESOURCES

Trusted support, communities and tools to lighten your load.

An Introduction to the Smilogie Method

The Smilogie Method offers a gentle, compassionate way to navigate the wobbles that come with cancer, hormones and everyday life. It invites you to pause, listen closely to your body and take small, mindful steps toward feeling more like yourself. It is built on the belief that healing does not need to be rushed and that even the smallest smile can soften the edges of a difficult day.

Each letter in S.M.I.L.O.G.I.E. is a guiding principle — not a rule — you can return to repeatedly. You will see the Smilogie Method woven throughout this book, quietly reminding you that even in the hardest times, small moments of peace can make a meaningful difference.

One small smile. One small shift.

One big change.

The Smilogie Method

Your Gentle Acronym for Change

Letter	Smilogie focus	Your gentle step
S	Smile	Soften the edges
M	Mindfulness	Meet this moment
I	Intuition	Identify your needs
L	Lifestyle	Listen with kindness
O	Optimism	Open to support
G	Gratitude	Ground yourself
I	Identity	Integrate who you are
E	Energy	Ease into balance

A Little Reflection

Each letter is a small step. Some days you may need one more than the others. ***Which letter do I need most today?*** Let that be your first step.

You have already begun, simply by pausing here.

1
A GENTLE REFRESHER

"I am more than my diagnosis."

Smilogie Moment

In my coaching work, I often hear a quiet whisper:
"I don't feel like myself anymore."
Whether it is cancer treatment, sudden menopause, or both, the wobble is real.
Each time, I offer the same gentle truth: **you are still you.**
Hormones may shake you, but they do not erase you.

A Gentle Note

If you have opened this book feeling unsure or overwhelmed, this first tab offers a calm, simple map of how breast and gynaecological cancers can shift hormones — and how those changes might feel in both body and mind.

Treatments and surgeries can flip hormones quickly. Mood, sleep, energy, intimacy, and even identity may wobble.

This is common — and it can be supported.

Take what helps, leave the rest, and choose one kind thing for yourself today.

A Small Hormone Refresher

When cancer treatment begins, it doesn't only target cells — it can touch your hormones too.

For many women, this means entering menopause suddenly, whether expected or not.

Here is a soft look at the main players:

Oestrogen

- Supports mood, bones, skin, vaginal comfort, and mental clarity.
- Treatments often lower or block oestrogen → **flushes, dryness, mood shifts, night sweats, bone changes**.

Progesterone

- Balances oestrogen, supports calm and sleep.
- Certain surgeries and treatments alter levels → **cycle changes, anxiety, sleep difficulties**.

Testosterone

- Fuels energy, confidence, focus, and intimacy.
- A dip may bring → **fatigue, low mood, and reduced desire**.

Thyroid

- Regulates energy and metabolism.
- Stress, inflammation, or treatment can shift function → **sluggishness, palpitations, anxiety, temperature swings**.

Cortisol

- Your stress hormone.
- Often rises with treatment or worry → **wired-but-tired feeling, poor sleep, emotional overwhelm**.

These changes are not a weakness.
They are biological shifts — and they can be supported.

SMILOGIE TIP

You do not need to track everything.

Choose *one* symptom — sleep, flushes, or energy — and gently notice what helps.

Small observations bring big clarity over time.

Hormones at a Glance

Hormone	What It Does	How Treatment Can Affect It
Oestrogen	Mood, bones, vaginal health, clarity	Often lowered/blocked → flushes, dryness, bone changes
Progesterone	Calm, sleep, balances oestrogen	Reduced → cycle & mood changes
Testosterone	Energy, confidence, intimacy	May decline → fatigue, low desire
Thyroid	Energy & metabolism	Stress/treatment may cause fatigue, weight/temp shifts
Cortisol	Stress response	↑ with worry/treatment → "wired but tired"

If you recognise yourself in these shifts, take a breath.

Your body is adapting — and support is possible.

A Look at Treatments & Hormone Shifts

Some treatments affect hormones directly; others do so indirectly.

This section keeps things simple and safe.

- **HRT (Hormone Replacement Therapy)**
  Often *not* recommended for breast or gynaecological cancers, though there are individual exceptions.
  Decisions are made with oncology + menopause teams.

- **Non-Hormonal Medications**
  Certain SSRIs/SNRIs, gabapentin, or clonidine may ease:
  √ hot flushes
  √ night sweats
  √ mood shifts or anxiety

  Ask your doctor if these might suit you.

- **Local (Vaginal) Supports**
  Moisturisers, lubricants, and in some cases **very low-dose vaginal oestrogen** may be considered — always check with your care team.

- **Lifestyle & Natural Supports**
  Gentle movement, nourishing meals, hydration, supplements, breathwork, mindfulness — small daily steps often make a noticeable difference.

SMILOGIE TIP

Ask your doctor:
"What are my safest options right now?"
One clear step forward is enough for today.

Non-Hormonal Supports — At a Glance

Type	Helps With	Examples (Always Check with Your Team)
Medications	Flushes, anxiety, sleep	SSRIs/SNRIs, gabapentin, clonidine
Vaginal Care	Dryness, discomfort	YES VM, SYLK, non-fragranced washes
Supplements	Energy, bones, mood	Omega-3, vitamin D, magnesium, probiotics
Lifestyle	Whole-body support	Hydration, gentle movement, pacing
Mind–Body	Anxiety, fear, sleep	Breathwork, mindfulness, journaling

Hormone Pathway at a Glance

Surgery / Chemotherapy / Radiotherapy / Hormone Therapy

↓

Changes in oestrogen, progesterone, testosterone, thyroid, cortisol

↓

Hot flushes • Dryness • Fatigue • Brain fog • Mood shifts

↓

Journaling • Hydration • Moisturisers • Movement • Supplements • Mindful pauses

Your symptoms are not random — they are connected, and they can be supported.

Bone & Heart Health Spotlight

When oestrogen dips, bones and heart sometimes need extra kindness:

- Ask about a **DEXA scan** and **cholesterol check**
- Add gentle weight-bearing movement
- Include calcium-rich foods + vitamin D
- Keep heart-care simple: hydration, balanced meals, stress pacing

  Small steps now protect your future self.

Fertility Spotlight

For younger women, cycles may pause or stop after treatment. Sometimes they return later.

- Ask early about egg preservation or fertility counselling
- Remember: **this is not your fault**
- Support exists — you don't have to work this out alone

Smilogie Self-Check

When everything feels like it's changing, pause gently:

Smile → soften your face

Breathe → slow inhale, long exhale

Notice → energy, mood, body

Choose → sleep? flushes? energy?

Act → one small step: water, rest, call your doctor

Interactive Prompt

Which hormone shift feels most noticeable in me right now?

What is one small thing I could try this week to soften that wobble?

A Gentle Refresher — At a Glance

Why It Matters

Cancer treatments can shift hormones suddenly. Understanding what's happening inside your body softens fear and builds steadiness.

Hormones & Their Roles

- Oestrogen → mood, skin, bones
- Progesterone → calm, sleep
- Testosterone → energy, desire
- Thyroid → metabolism, energy
- Cortisol → stress response

Quick Supports

- Track one symptom at a time
- Hydrate
- Move gently
- Use moisturisers/lubricants as needed
- Routinely check in with your doctor
- Journal or practise Smilogie Sparks for calm

Closing Reflection

When you understand what is happening in your body, the wobbles lose their power.

Knowledge softens fear; small steps build steadiness.

Gentle Prompt

What small shift will I try this week — rest, hydration, movement, or simply a soft smile?

2
TREATMENT & HORMONES

"Knowledge softens fear"

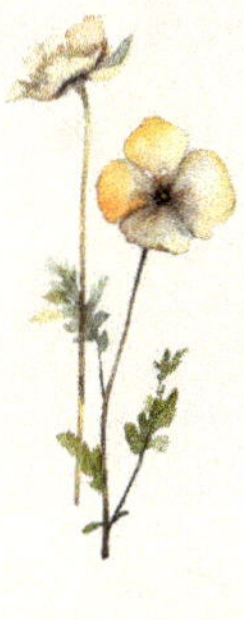

Smilogie Moment

A woman once said to me, "They explained the treatment... but not how it would make me feel as a woman." That stayed with me. Understanding treatment is not only science—it's also making sense of the wobbles it creates in everyday life.

A Gentle Note

Cancer care can be a lot—surgery, chemo, radiotherapy, tablets—and the side-effect lists are long. What is less often explained is how these treatments shift your hormones, and why that can change energy, sleep, mood, libido, and even how "you" feel in your own skin.

This section offers a calm overview of how each treatment may affect hormones and why the changes you notice are real—not imagined—and supportable. Take what helps, leave the rest, and meet yourself with compassion as you read.

A Gentle Overview

- **Surgery (ovaries, uterus, or breast)** → Can trigger sudden menopause. Symptoms may arrive quickly — hot flushes, mood shifts, or changes in cycles if you still had them

- **Chemotherapy** → Often leads to treatment-induced menopause. Wobbles may include hot flushes, night sweats, fatigue, brain fog, and dryness

- **Radiotherapy** → Depending on the area treated, it may not directly affect hormones, but it can stress the body and influence cycles, energy, and rest

- **Hormone Therapy (Tamoxifen, Aromatase Inhibitors, etc.)** → Designed to block or lower oestrogen. They help protect against recurrence but may bring symptoms like hot flushes, joint aches, vaginal dryness, or bone changes

Every woman responds differently. Your experience is unique — and it is valid.

Targeted & Immunotherapy Note

Some women also receive targeted therapies (e.g. Herceptin, CDK4/6 inhibitors) or immunotherapy.

These do not usually alter hormones directly, but can contribute to fatigue, joint aches, or cycle changes.

Always note how you feel and share updates with your healthcare team.

Hormone Shifts at a Glance

Treatment	Hormone Effect	Common Wobbles
Surgery (ovaries / uterus)	Sudden drop in oestrogen & progesterone	Hot flushes, night sweats, mood changes
Chemotherapy	Induced menopause, lowers oestrogen / testosterone	Fatigue, brain fog, dryness
Radiotherapy	Indirect effect via stress on body / ovaries	Cycle changes, exhaustion, sleep disruption
Hormone Therapy (Tamoxifen / AIs)	Blocks or lowers oestrogen	Hot flushes, joint aches, vaginal dryness, bone changes

Spotlight on Hormone Therapy

- **Tamoxifen** → Blocks oestrogen in breast tissue → flushes, mood changes, dryness.

- **Aromatase Inhibitors (letrozole, anastrozole, exemestane)** → Reduce oestrogen production → joint stiffness, bone changes, fatigue.

Ask about bone scans, weight-bearing exercise, vitamin D, calcium, and supportive medicines if needed.

Some side effects fade with time; others need ongoing support.

SMILOGIE TIP

If you are unsure, ask: *"Is this likely to ease, or should we look at supports now?"*

Steroid Spotlight

Steroids are often given alongside chemotherapy. They can bring short-term wobbles such as poor sleep, extra appetite, or mood swings.

These are treatment effects, not weakness — and they usually pass once steroids are stopped.

Fertility Note

If fertility or family planning is on your mind—before, during, or after treatment—your team can talk through options (e.g., preservation, timing, early-menopause supports). It is okay if you are not sure what you want yet; questions are a good start.

Evidence Nugget

Hormone therapy reduces recurrence risk and improves outcomes for many women — but personalisation is key *(ASCO 2023)*.

When to Call Your Doctor

Most side effects are manageable, but contact your care team if anything feels worrying or disrupts daily life.

Call promptly if you notice:

- Unexplained bleeding or sudden, severe pain
- Swelling, redness, or warmth in a limb (possible clot)
- Shortness of breath, chest pain, or dizziness
- Any side effect so strong it limits your day-to-day life

Your safety matters. No concern is too small.

Smilogie Lens on Treatment

M – Mindfulness → Pause before appointments, breathe, and notice how you feel.

I – Intuition → Observe which side effects bother you most — they matter.

L – Lifestyle → Hydration, rest, and balanced meals help steady hormonal shifts.

G – Gratitude → Name one thing your body is still doing well — it shifts perspective.

Smilogie Support in Practice

- **Keep a Symptom Journal** → Track what changes, what helps, what worsens.
- **Anchor Yourself at Appointments** → Bring notes or a trusted listener.
- **Prepare Small Comforts** → Cooling scarf for flushes, soothing tea for digestion, soft blanket for fatigue.
- **Explore Complementary Supports** → Physiotherapy, oncology massage, acupuncture, or evidence-based approaches like CBT or mindfulness for flushes and anxiety — always check with your oncology team first.
- **Ask for Clarification** → No question is too small; your doctor works for you.

My Treatment & Hormone Tracker

Even notitng one or two words — "tired," "foggy," "better after walk" — builds clarity over time.

Date ....

Treatment / Medication ....

....

....

Body Wobbles ....

....

....

Mind / Heart Wobbles ....

....

....

What Helped Today ....

....

....

....

Smilogie Reminder

These shifts are not your fault.
They are your body's response to treatment.
You deserve compassion as you move through them.

Date ....

Treatment / Medication ....

....

....

Body Wobbles ....

....

....

....

Mind / Heart Wobbles ....

....

....

....

What Helped Today ....

....

....

....

SMILOGIE TIP

When side effects appear, jot them in a small notebook and bring them to your next appointment.

It helps you feel clear and confident — and ensures your care team understands your real-life experience.

Treatment & Hormones — at a Glance

Why It Matters

Different treatments influence hormones in different ways.

The wobbles you feel are real, not imagined.

Understanding what is happening softens fear and guides you toward support.

Treatment Effects

Treatment	Hormone Effect	Common Wobbles
Surgery (ovaries / uterus)	Sudden drop in oestrogen & progesterone	Hot flushes, mood changes, night sweats
Chemotherapy	Induces menopause, lowers oestrogen / testosterone	Fatigue, brain fog, dryness
Radiotherapy	Indirect stress on ovaries / body	Cycle changes, exhaustion, poor sleep
Hormone Therapy (Tamoxifen / AIs)	Blocks or lowers oestrogen	Hot flushes, joint aches, dryness, bone changes

Smilogie Reminders

- Track how you feel — even one word helps.
- Bring your notes to appointments — clarity is kindness.
- Your body is responding to treatment — not failing you.

Quick Supports

- Cooling scarf for flushes.
- Journaling for clarity.
- Soothing teas or warm broths.
- Stretching for joint aches.
- Guilt-free rest.

Closing Reflection

Understanding how treatment and hormones interact removes some of the mystery — and with it, some of the fear.

Clarity creates room for kindness and self-trust.

Gentle Prompt

Which treatment effect feels most noticeable right now?

What is one small support I can try today?

3
DOCTOR VISITS

"Clarity is kindness to yourself."

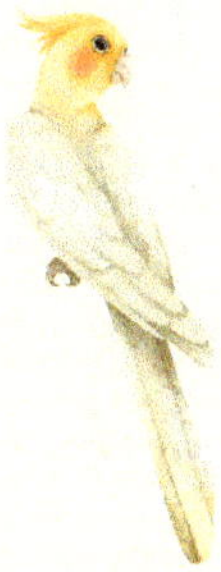

Personal Message

I used to arrive at appointments with my mind racing — and leave having forgotten half of what I meant to ask.

Frustrated, I began carrying a small notebook with my key questions and brief symptom notes.

That simple habit brought back my confidence — and a quiet sense of control.

A Gentle Note

Doctor visits can feel overwhelming. With so much information, the most important questions can slip away.

This section helps you prepare so you leave with answers — and calm.

It is okay to feel nervous or rushed; many women do.

You deserve the time to be heard.

Before Your Appointment

List the following:

- **Current medicines / supplements** (and any allergies) — show this first.

- **Top 3 questions** — one line each.

- **Symptom snapshot** — what, when, what helped.

Digital supports

If paper is not your thing, open your phone's Notes app or record a short voice memo for questions and symptoms.

Take photos of medication boxes or scan appointment letters to keep everything in one place.

If you need extra time, an interpreter, or a support person — ask ahead.

You are allowed to.

Smilogie Spark

Confidence often begins with a single clear question.

Questions You Might Ask

(Pick three that feel most relevant.)

- What are my options for this symptom — and what are the pros / cons?
- Are there non-hormonal or local (vaginal) supports I can try?
- How might this treatment affect my hormones long-term?
- What red-flag symptoms mean I should call you or urgent care?
- Can we plan bone / heart checks (DEXA, vitamin D, lipids) if needed?
- Are there targeted / immunotherapies or physio / psycho-oncology supports I should know about?
- What should I track between now and our next visit?

If English is not your first language or you process information slowly, you can ask for written summaries, extra time, or an interpreter.

> Asking does not make you a burden — it helps your care team help you.

During Your Appointment

(some micro-scripts)

- "Could you explain that in everyday words?"
- "What is the one thing you'd like me to do first?"
- "Can we write the plan in 3 steps?"
- "What should improve by when... and what if it doesn't?"

After Your Appointment – Two-Minute Debrief

My plan in 3 steps

....

....

....

What to watch / who to call

1. ....
2. ....
3. ....

Follow-ups booked

Date Time

....

....

....

....

One feeling I'm leaving with

Doctor Visit Notes

- Questions I want to ask

- Side effects or symptoms I have noticed

- What helped (even a little)

- Notes from today's visit

- How I feel after this visit: relieved / hopeful / unsure

- Red flags & who to contact

- Next appointments / tests

Treatment / Side-Effect Tracker

Date | Treatment/Medicine | Body wobbles | Mind/heart wobbles | What I tried | Helped?

Even one or two words — "foggy," "better after walk" — build valuable insight over time.

Medicines & Supplements Log Safety Note

Name & Dose

Why I Take It

Start Date

Timing & Notes

....

....

....

....

....

....

Checked with Team (√)

....

....

....

....

....

....

....

Check for interactions and timing, especially during active chemotherapy or radiotherapy.

Product names in this book are examples, not endorsements — always choose with your healthcare team.

Scan-xiety Mini-Plan

(Use whenever scan day nerves appear.)

1. **Name it:** "This is scan-xiety."
2. **Set a worry window:** 10–15 minutes per day — write, then close the notebook.
3. **Plan a post-scan ritual:** a walk, a coffee, or time with a friend.
4. **If / Then card:** If a new symptom lasts > 48–72 hours → I call

Smilogie Lens for Appointments

S – Smile → Soften your face, even in the waiting room.
M – Mindfulness → Take one slow breath before speaking.
I – Intuition → Write down the question that feels most important, even if it seems small.
L – Listen → Repeat back what you've heard to be sure you understood.

Doctor Visits — At a Glance

Why It Matters

Prepared questions + simple notes = calmer visits, clearer plans.

Quick Supports

Top-3 questions • Symptom snapshot • Teach-back • Two-minute debrief • Tear-out trackers

SMILOGIE ADVOCACY SCRIPT

"Doctor, this side effect is affecting my daily life — what are my options?"

Affirmation

Clarity is kindness to myself.

SMILOGIE TIP

If you forgot to ask, message the clinic afterwards with one concise question — it still counts.

Reminder

No question is too small.
If it matters to you, it matters.

Closing Reflection

Prepared voices are heard.
Your questions are acts of self-care, not confrontation.

Gentle Prompt

What is the one question I'll bring to my next appointment?
Write it down now.

4
BODY WOBBLES

"I listen to my body with kindness"

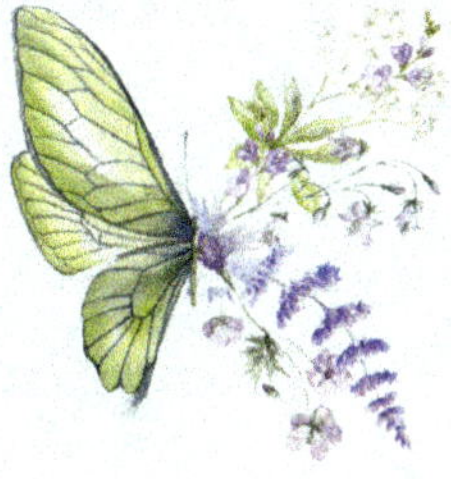

Smilogie Moment

There was a time my body felt like it belonged to someone else — tired, achy, unfamiliar.

A friend once said, "I don't trust my body anymore; it keeps surprising me."

I knew what she meant.

Cancer treatment and hormone shifts can bring waves of new sensations.

What I have learned is this: your body is still on your side.

Listening with kindness can turn frustration into softer care.

A Gentle Note

Treatment can make your body feel unrecognisable — hot flushes, night sweats, joint aches, dryness, fatigue.

These wobbles are real and exhausting.

This section will not list *everything*; but it does offer clear, simple supports and reassurance.

Your body is responding to powerful changes. With small, steady steps and compassion, you can ease the edges and feel more at home in yourself again.

Common Body Wobbles

You may not experience all of these — and you do not have to read them all at once. Dip in as needed.

Wobble	What's Happening	Gentle Supports
Hot Flushes & Night Sweats	Sudden waves of heat	Cooling layers, fans, paced breathing (4 in / 6 out), spot triggers (warm rooms, caffeine, alcohol, spicy food).
Vaginal Dryness & Discomfort	Lower oestrogen	Moisturisers (YES VM), lubricants (YES / SYLK), fragrance-free wash, cotton underwear. Discuss with your clinician.
Joint & Muscle Aches (AIs / Tamoxifen)	Hormonal shifts + medication	Gentle mobility, warmth, light strength work, magnesium (if approved). Ask about med alternatives if severe.

Fatigue	Deep tiredness not fixed by sleep	Pacing, rest before crash, brief naps (10–20 min), hydration, protein + fibre snacks.
Bone Health	Oestrogen dip → density change	Ask about DEXA scan, calcium-rich foods, vitamin D (if advised), weight-bearing exercise.
Skin & Hair Changes	Dryness, thinning, tenderness	Barrier skincare, SPF, soft natural fabrics, gentle headwear.
Digestive Wobbles	Constipation, bloating, reflux	Fluids, warm drinks, gradual fibre (prunes / chia / kiwi), bland broths for diarrhoea, smaller meals for reflux.
Lymph	Swelling, heaviness, skin warmth / colour change	Change to Physio or Lymphoedema clinic referral. Compression if prescribed.
Neuropathy	Tingling / numb hands or feet	Non-slip shoes, clear floors, moisturise daily, ask team re: therapies.

Urinary / Bladder Changes	Frequency, urgency, UTIs	Hydration, vaginal moisturiser, pelvic-floor relaxation, wee after intimacy; see GP if persistent.
Mouth & Taste Changes	Dry mouth, sores	Lukewarm foods, sauces, soft toothbrush, saline / bicarb rinse, alcohol-free mouthwash.
Headaches / Migraines	Hormone shifts / stress / dehydration	Hydrate, regular meals, shoulder mobility, dark quiet rest, magnesium (if approved).
Light-headedness / Dizziness	Dehydration, anaemia, meds	Rise slowly, sip fluids, sit to dress, tell your team if persistent.
Axillary Web (Cording)	Tight bands after node surgery	Gentle mobility, early physio input.
Hand–Foot / Nail Care	Tender palms / soles, nail ridges	Fragrance-free emollients, cool soaks, cotton socks, cautious nail care; report pain or infection.

Integrative Supports

- **Acupuncture** — may ease flushes, joint pain, or neuropathy.
- **Oncology Massage / Reflexology** — relaxation, pain relief, circulation (check with team first).
- **CBT-I** — cognitive behavioural therapy for insomnia; proven for cancer-related sleep issues. Ask if offered locally or online.

Cooling & Comfort Kit

- Handheld / neck fan
- Cooling pillow
- Cotton / linen layers (+ spare night top)
- Water bottle
- Peppermint or fennel tea
- Moisturiser / lubricant sachets
- Heat pack • Soft socks

Micro Mobility (60–90 Seconds)

(Little and often beats all-at-once.)

- Neck circles × 3
- Shoulder rolls + chest opener × 5
- Ankle pumps / calf raises × 10

Pelvic & Intimacy Care

- Moisturiser routine (3–4× per week or as advised).
- Lubricant for intimacy.
- Pelvic floor: learn to relax as well as strengthen (long, slow exhales).
- Pelvic health physiotherapy for scars, prolapse, leakage or pain.
- If penetration is painful → ask about physio and, if approved, gentle dilator use with lube + breath-led relaxation.

Skin Barrier Basics (Radiation & Beyond)

- Mild fragrance-free cleanser
- Pat dry
- Hydrate → moisturise → occlusive at night for dry spots
- Daily SPF
- Soft natural fabrics.
- Scar Care & Adhesions (when fully healed): moisturise with unscented lotion; slow circular massage around scars; gentle stretching. Ask physio for safe techniques.

Smilogie Body-Scan (1 Minute)

Smile softly → Scan head to toe: "Where is the loudest wobble?" → Soothe that spot → Whisper: "Thank you, body — message received."

Your Wobble Flare Plan

(Journal box for repeated use.)

My early signs

....

Likely triggers

....

My 3 steps

1. ....
2. ....
3. ....

Who I tell / when I call

....

....

....

....

Pattern Tracking

Wobbles often have triggers — stress, certain foods, time of day.

Jotting patterns helps you and your team see links; sometimes the smallest tweak brings real relief.

Body Kindness Rituals

Warm bath + slow moisturising afterwards

- Gentle stretch or child's pose
- Soft blanket + tea + three long exhales
- Step outside for 3 minutes of fresh air and sunlight.

Body Kindness Card

Keep a pocket reminder (or phone note):

- "This is my body's way of healing."
- "I am listening with kindness."
- "This wobble will pass."

SMILOGIE TIP

If flares follow "good days," try the 80 % rule — stop at 80% of your energy so you have some left for healing.

Body Wobbles Through the Smilogie Lens

S – Smile → Soften your face; calm your system.
M – Mindfulness → Notice one body message.
I – Intuition → Ask: movement, rest, or soothing touch?
L – Lifestyle → Hydrate, move gently, moisturise, breathe.
O – Openness → Try one new support (fan, lube, mobility snack).
G – Gratitude → Thank one part of your body today.
I – Identity → Your symptoms don't define you.
E – Energy → Pace it like a budget, not an overdraft.

Safety Check — Call Your Team If …

If in doubt, call early — you don't have to "wait and see."

- Fever or infection signs during treatment → urgent.
- New or worsening one-sided swelling, redness, or limb pain.
- Shortness of breath, chest pain, fainting, rapid heartbeat.
- Wounds not healing.
- Severe / new bone pain, spreading numbness or weakness.
- Digestive issues that don't settle or sudden weight loss.
- Any wobble that feels very different or frightening.

At a Glance

- The most common wobbles are fatigue, flushes, dryness, and aches — you are not alone in them.
- Small supports add up: one cool sip, one stretch, one rest.

Affirmation

"My body is healing in its own rhythm, and I honour that."

Smilogie Reminder

Your body is not failing you — it is working hard every day. Each wobble is a message asking for understanding.
(Aligned with Macmillan and EONS symptom-support guidelines.)

Closing Reflection

Your body may feel different, but it is still yours.

Meeting it with kindness can transform frustration into connection.

Gentle Prompt

Which body wobble feels most present right now?

SMILOGIE TIP

When a wobble appears, ask yourself, "What is the kindest response I can give my body right now?" Sometimes it's movement, sometimes rest, sometimes acceptance. If unsure, call anyway. You are not "bothering" anyone.

5
MIND WOBBLES

"I give my mind moments of calm."

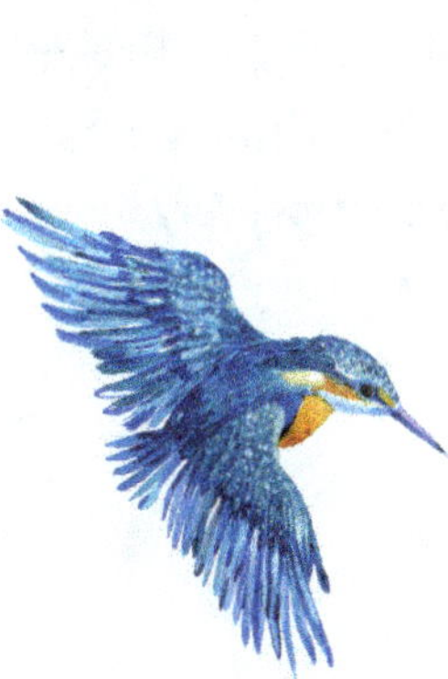

Smilogie Moment

There was a time when my mind felt like a runaway train — racing at night, foggy by day, whispering "what if?"

Many of the women I support say the same: "I can't switch my mind off."

What I have learned is this: we do not have to silence the mind.

We can offer it small, steady anchors of calm.

A Gentle Note

Cancer and hormone shifts can make the mind wobble — fear of recurrence, pre-appointment nerves, brain fog, or simply not feeling like "you."

Sometimes, after treatment, the mind holds imprints — flashbacks, sudden surges of fear, a readiness to brace even when life seems quiet.

These are not failings; they are signs of how much you've been through — and they respond to gentleness.

Your mind deserves the same care as your body.

You do not need to control every thought; an invitation to pause, breathe, and try one tiny calming ritual is enough for today.

Common Mind Wobbles

Wobble	Why It Happens	Gentle Supports
Anxiety / Fear	Stress, uncertainty, trauma	Slow breathing, grounding, guided relaxation
Brain Fog	Chemo, menopause, fatigue	Short lists, single-tasking, patience
Sleep Worries	Stress, flushes, hormone shifts	Bedtime ritual, screen-free wind-down, herbal or ginger tea
Identity Shifts	Hormonal + cancer changes	Journaling, affirmations, creativity, safe connection
Scan-xiety	Anticipation, past trauma	Grounding breathwork, supportive companion, soothing ritual
Friendship Drift / Social Overwhelm	Changing comfort levels	"Low-lift" contact — voice note, brief walk, no-pressure text
Parenting while Healing	Balancing care for others + self	Micro-rituals, child-friendly scripts, ask for practical help

Mind Wobbles Through the Smilogie Lens

M – Mindfulness → Pause for three slow breaths.

I – Intuition → Ask: Does my mind need rest, expression, or gentle distraction?

G – Gratitude → Name three tiny things you're thankful for.

E – Energy → Protect mental energy; step back from overstimulation or endless scrolling.

Thought-Reset Rituals

- Write a worry, then fold or tear it away.
- Cool cloth on forehead = pause signal.
- Soft smile in the mirror — even if it feels shaky.
- "Worry Window" → choose a 10–15 min slot later; let your mind rest in preparation.
- 5-4-3-2-1 Grounding → notice 5 things you see, 4 touch, 3 hear, 2 smell, 1 taste.

Smilogie Worry-Window Card

(Copy into diary or phone notes.)

Today's Window

Time ....

Place ....

If a worry appears before then → jot it here

....

....

....

....

....

and remind yourself → "I'll come back to you at my window."

When the window closes → fold paper / close note → do one soothing thing (walk, stretch, music, tea).

Reminder

You do not have to carry every thought all day. Your mind is allowed to rest outside the window.

"One woman told me she keeps her Worry-Window card in her pocket on scan days."

Creative Calm

Sometimes peace arrives through gentle expression, not stillness: colour a mandala, knit or crochet, listen to music, write a short poem, doodle in a margin.

A small creative act can turn restless energy into something soft and healing.

The 60-Second Smilogie Reset

Smile softly → Breathe in 4 through the nose, exhale 6 through the mouth → Say silently, "I am safe right now." → Sip water.

Even one minute can interrupt the spiral and bring you back to the present.

Community & Connection

Isolation can make wobbles louder; sharing them softens their hold.

- Join a gentle support group (online or local).
- Reach out to one trusted friend or family member.
- Share one worry aloud — it often feels lighter.

Some women keep a photo of a supportive friend in their pocket — a quiet anchor of calm.

Information Boundaries

- Choose one trusted update source.
- Batch medical admin into a weekly "paperwork hour."
- Mute doom-scroll triggers.
- Replace late-night searching with a "questions-for-clinic" note.

Post-Cancer Imprints

Sometimes the body and mind keep "imprints" of what you've lived through — a sudden jolt, vivid memory, or feeling on alert even when you're safe.

This is not regression, it is a normal trauma response that can heal with support.

Gentle, evidence-based options include:

- **EMDR / Somatic Therapies** → help the body and brain file away distressing memories.
- **CBT-I** → structured tools that restore sleep after treatment-related insomnia.
- **MBSR / CBT** → mindfulness-based and cognitive approaches proven to reduce anxiety.

You do not have to face this alone — these therapies exist to help your mind feel safe again.

Evidence Nugget

A 2019 meta-analysis found CBT-I improved sleep for around 70 % of cancer survivors.

Parenting & Caring While Healing

Simple Scripts

- "My tiredness isn't your fault. Your job is play and school; my job is rest and care."
- "I can listen for five minutes now; then I'll rest, and we can read later."

Micro-Rituals

- Ten-minute floor-time.
- Shared song at bedtime.
- Soothing hot drinks together after school.

Mind Wobbles — At a Glance

Why It Matters

Cancer does not just affect the body — it leaves footprints in the mind.

Anxiety, fog, and fear are *normal responses*, not failings.

Smilogie Reminders

- You are not your thoughts.
- Pausing brings calm.
- A soft smile can interrupt a spiral.

Quick Supports

- Three slow breaths.
- Write one worry, then let it go.
- Five-senses grounding.
- Guided apps → Calm • Insight Timer • Headspace.
- Talk with someone you trust.

Evidence Nugget

Seek professional help if the spirals feel too strong — cognitive-behavioural and mindfulness practices meaningfully reduce cancer-related anxiety (*Psycho-Oncology* 2021).

SMILOGIE TIP

Your thoughts don't need to be controlled — only cared for.

Even a single moment of calm can change the tone of your day.

Smilogie Reminder

You are not your thoughts.

They may wobble — but you remain steady underneath.

Closing Reflection

Your mind deserves gentleness, not pressure.

Giving yourself permission to pause, breathe, and soften your inner voice is an act of strength.

Gentle Prompt

Which letter of S M I L O G I E could help my mind today — M for Mindfulness, G for Gratitude, or E for Energy?

6
HEART WOBBLES

"My heart deserves gentleness."

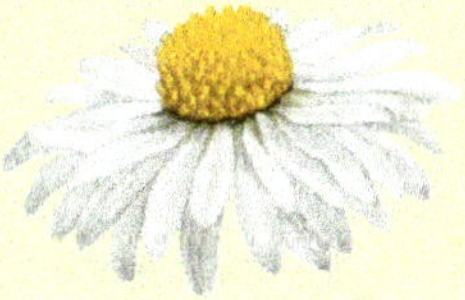

Smilogie Moment

A woman once said to me, “I was prepared for treatment — not for what it would do to my relationships.”

Cancer can touch closeness, identity, fertility, and even trust in your own body.

I have felt my own heart wobble through life’s shifts, and learned this:
the heart often needs the most gentleness — and we offer it the least.

A Gentle Note

Cancer does not only affect the body and mind — it touches the heart.

Intimacy may change. Relationships may wobble. Grief may surface for what feels altered or lost.

Sudden or early menopause after treatment can add layers to mood, desire, and closeness. This is biology, not personal failure. You deserve thoughtful support — and if things feel difficult, an oncology-aware menopause specialist can be effective.

Your heart may feel fragile, but it is also deeply resilient.

With small honesty, soft connection, and simple ritual, steadiness returns.

A Voice from Another Woman

"I thought intimacy was over for us.

We started with a 30-second hug every evening.

It sounds so small, but it changed how we faced everything."

A First-Day Friendly Note

If you only remember one thing, let it be this:

- **You deserve comfort and connection.**

Start tiny

1. One honest conversation.
2. One gentle ritual of closeness (a bedtime tea check-in).
3. Ask for help sooner than you think you "should."

Common Heart Wobbles

- **Relationship shifts** → Roles may change; friends may not know what to say.
  Small, honest conversations reduce tension.

- **Intimacy changes** → Body image, dryness, low libido, pain.
  Safety, slowness, and clear communication rebuild confidence.

- **Fertility grief** → Mourning what might not be.
  Naming the grief is part of healing.

- **Isolation** → Feeling different or misunderstood.
  One safe person can soften the load.

- **Loss & layered grief** → Loss of ease, normality, or safety.
  Acknowledging it makes space for recovery.

- **Care-partner strain** → Carers may feel stretched too.
  Boundaries + shared planning lighten the load.

- **Friendship drift** → Some step back; you may feel left behind.
  Low-lift contact helps: a voice note, a short walk, a "thinking of you."

- **Parenting pressure** → Limited energy + children's needs.
  Micro-rituals and simple scripts support connection.

Quick Check-In

(No right answer — noticing is the first kindness.)

Today I feel...

- ☐ Closed-off
- ☐ Tender but willing
- ☐ Open to closeness

Intimacy Care at a Glance

Dryness & Discomfort

- Regular vaginal moisturisers (YES VM) + water- or plant-based lubricants (YES, SYLK).
- Avoid fragranced washes. Cotton underwear helps.

Pain or Burning (GSM / Entry Pain)

- Go slowly; use generous lubricant.
- Long, slow exhales relax the pelvic floor.
- Ask about pelvic-floor physio or gentle graded dilators.
- Some women benefit from topical lidocaine 2–5% applied 10–15 minutes before intimacy.

Lower Desire

- Common with hormone shifts, fatigue, and mood.
- Desire often follows **comfort + time + no pressure**.

Body Confidence

- Soft lighting, fabrics you like, mirror-kindness, focus on sensation over appearance.
- Grief about changes is allowed — and so is pleasure.

EVIDENCE NUGGET

Even small affectionate touch — a hug, a hand-hold — can lower stress hormones and strengthen connection.

Responsive Desire 101

It is normal not to feel desire at the start.

Desire often appears *after* you feel safe, relaxed, and gently engaged.

Recipe:

Comfort + time + no pressure + pleasant sensations → desire may follow.

Start with a cuddle, warmth, music, or gentle massage, then follow what feels right.

Consent & Communication Micro-Scripts

- "I want closeness, and I also need comfort. Can we go slowly and check in as we go?"
- "Can we slow down and try more lubricant?"
- "I want connection, not sex today. Could we walk, read, or curl up together?"
- "Thank you for being gentle with me."

Nothing is "too small" to mention. Your comfort matters.

Green / Yellow / Red Check-In:

- **Green** = open
- **Yellow** = gentle only
- **Red** = need space

Rupture → Repair

Name it → own your part → reset with a hug + five-minute talk. Frequent small repairs keep relationships strong.

Tiny Couple Rituals (3 minutes)

- **Tea Check-In** → 5 minutes each, uninterrupted.
- **Repair Hug** → 30-second hug after an argument.
- **Weekly "Good Things" List** → each shares one appreciation.

Body Kindness & Confidence

- **Body neutrality:** "My body is my home; it doesn't need to be perfect to be worthy."
- **Mirror moments:** Ten seconds. Soft smile. One thing you appreciate.
- **Thank-you letters:** Write to a body part that carried you through.
- **Sensation-first:** Focus on comfort, warmth, touch — not appearance.

Closeness includes partner intimacy, friendship touch, or reconnecting gently with yourself.

For Loved Ones

Ask:

"Would you like advice, help, or just company?"

Often, what helps most is something small and steady:

a short message ("thinking of you")

a practical offer ("I'm at the shop — need milk?")

quiet company without needing to talk

Avoid comparisons.

Avoid forced positivity.

If you or your partner ever feel persistently overwhelmed, trapped, or unsafe, reach out to your healthcare team.

You deserve care, safety, and support.

One-Minute Heart Reset

Smile softly → one slow breath → whisper "I am safe and loved."

Place a hand over your heart and feel three beats.

(Aligned with British Menopause Society & ESMO Survivorship guidance.)

Heart Wobbles Through the Smilogie Lens

S – Smile → Softens tension; opens the door to connection.

M – Mindfulness → One slow breath before a hard conversation.

O – Openness → Say what you need, ask for help, allow closeness on your terms.

G – Gratitude → Name one thing you appreciate about your body, partner, or friend.

E – Energy → Protect emotional energy; rest before big talks.

SMILOGIE TIP

Relationships are not built on perfection — they are built on presence.

Showing up gently, even when you wobble, is enough.

Smilogie Reminder

You are lovable as you are — with scars, shifts, and all.
Your heart deserves tenderness, always.

Reflection & Tiny First Step

The heart carries so much — love, grief, longing, hope.

When you meet these feelings with gentleness instead of judgement, healing begins.

Tiny First Step

Tonight, give your heart one soft minute — a breath, a hand-to-heart touch, or a quiet "thank you" for all it has carried.

Gentle Prompt

Which heart wobble feels most tender for me right now?

What is one small act of gentleness I can offer my heart today?

7
NURTURE & NUTRITION

"Nourishment is an act of self-love."

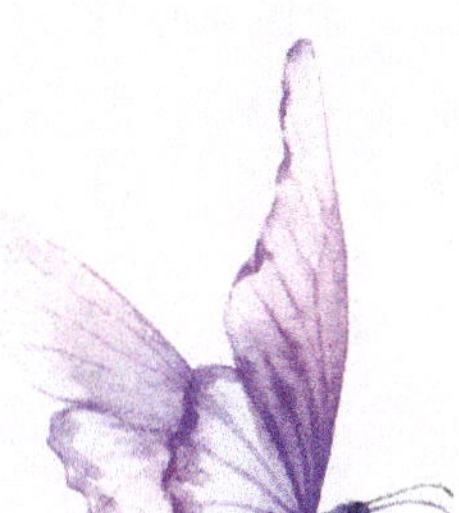

Smilogie Moment

A woman once whispered, "I feel guilty for not eating perfectly since my diagnosis."

I smiled and said, "Perfection isn't nourishment — kindness is."

In my own wobbles, I learned that food, water, and tiny rituals were not just fuel —

they were love notes to my body.

Even one slow sip of water can be a quiet act of care.

A Gentle Note

Treatment and hormone changes can shift everything — appetite, taste, digestion, energy.

You may crave comfort foods or have no interest in cooking. **That is human**.

This tab is not about rules.

It is about remembering that **eating is also healing** — physically and emotionally.

Let hydration, warm meals, and little rituals bring steadiness back to your days.

Smilogie Spark

Every calm bite tells your nervous system, "You're safe."

First-Day Friendly Note

If you remember only one thing:

Water + Protein + Colour

Start simple today:

- a full glass of water
- one small source of protein
- a splash of natural colour (berries, greens, herbs, fruit)

That is enough.

Nurture & Nutrition Essentials

Hydration — Your Quiet Ally

Hydration supports energy, bowels, temperature, and skin.

Herbal teas, diluted juices, and broths count.

If you are flushing, sweating, or have diarrhoea, ask your team about safe electrolytes.

The Smilogie Plate — Balance, Not Rules

Think **1–2–3** at each meal:

1. **Protein** — eggs, beans, tofu, yoghurt, fish, chicken
2. **Plants** — vegetables + fruit
3. **Comfort Extras** — healthy fats, fibre, flavour

Pair carbohydrates with protein or fat for steadier mood and energy.

Pause halfway through eating and check in with your body: *"How do I feel?"*

Gentle Digestion Support

- Warm, soft meals soothe better than raw or crunchy.
- Constipation → fluids + gradual fibre (chia, prunes, oats).
- Loose stools → binding foods (banana, rice, toast).
- Reflux → smaller meals; stay upright after eating.

Protein for Repair

Include a little protein at every meal — eggs, lentils, yoghurt, tofu, fish, nuts/nut butters.

Supports recovery, skin, hair, immune strength, and stamina.

Healthy Fats for Hormone Calm

Nuts, seeds, avocado, olive oil, and oily fish ease dryness and support mood and brain health.

Bone & Heart Kindness

- Calcium-rich foods + vitamin D (if advised)
- Gentle weight-bearing movement (walking, light resistance)
- Colourful plants and omega-3s support heart health

Even a 5-minute walk after meals aids digestion and circulation.

Evidence Nugget

Balanced protein + hydration during treatment supports energy and tissue repair (Clinical Nutrition 2022).

Comfort Counts

Your favourite soup, a warm drink, or a square of chocolate are not "cheats."

They are **comfort medicine for the heart**.

Golden Milk — The Smilogie Evening Elixir

Warm milk (plant or dairy) +
½ tsp turmeric + pinch cinnamon + dash ginger + crack of black pepper.
Optional: honey or vanilla *after* heating.
Sip slowly under a blanket.

Supports digestion, joints, and relaxation — but mostly, it is **a hug in a cup**.

Four Modern Nurture Boosters

1. **Gratitude Bite** → Pause over your first mouthful: "Thank you, body."
2. **Gentle Gut Care** → prebiotics (oats, leeks, onions, apples); safe probiotics if advised.
3. **Anti-inflammatory Allies** → turmeric, ginger, cinnamon, berries.
4. **Mindful Eating Moments** → sit down, slow down, breathe between bites.

Smilogie Pantry & 5-Minute Meals

Nourishment Basket → oatcakes, nut butter, dark chocolate, herbal teas
Freezer Friends → soups, vegetable mixes, bread, frozen fruit for smoothies

5-minute ideas:

- Toast + avocado + egg
- Yoghurt + chia + berries
- Tinned salmon + lemon + crackers
- Grains + chickpeas + olive oil
- Lentil soup + cheese + olive oil drizzle

Symptom-Smart Eating

Choose what fits **today**:

Wobble	Gentle Helps
Nausea	Cold foods, dry crackers, ginger tea
Taste changes	Plastic cutlery, marinades, chilled foods
Mouth sores / dry mouth	Soft, moist foods; baking-soda rinse
Constipation	Fluids, warm drinks, slow fibre
Diarrhoea	BRAT foods, broths, electrolytes
Reflux	Small meals, upright posture
Appetite loss	Smoothies, snack meals, calorie-dense extras
Steroid hungries	Pair carbs with protein/fat; structured snacks

Safety & Good to Know

- Always check supplements with your oncology or dietitian team.
- Some herbs interact with treatment — confirm before use.
- Whole-soy foods ≠ high-dose soy supplements; clarify with your team.
- During low immunity, follow food-safety guidance carefully.
- If unsure, ask for a referral to a **registered oncology dietitian**.

Clinician Integration Note

This tab aligns with major oncology-nutrition guidelines (WCRF/AICR, EONS).

Clinicians may share excerpts in patient-education settings with attribution.

Gentle Nurture Rituals

- Drink a glass of water mindfully on waking.
- Light a candle at meals to create calm.
- Keep fruit and nuts within easy reach.
- Enjoy Golden Milk as a signal to rest.
- Pair nourishment with gentle movement — a 5-minute stretch or walk.

Smilogie Spark

One soothing bowl + one slow breath = a recipe for peace.

Pocket Self-Check Box

(Any one tick is enough today.)

Today I gave my body one kind thing:

- ☐ A full glass of water
- ☐ A colourful plate
- ☐ A slow, mindful bite
- ☐ A Golden Milk moment
- ☐ A breath of gratitude

Nurture Through the Smilogie Lens

L – Lifestyle → one soothing daily ritual

O – Openness → try one gentle new food this week

G – Gratitude → pause before meals: "Thank you, body."

E – Energy → choose foods that lift, not drain

One-Minute Nourish Reset

Smile softly → sip water → ask:

"What would feel kind right now — a snack, a stretch, or stillness?"

Do that one thing.

Smilogie Reminder

Food is not only fuel — it is **comfort, connection, and care**.

Each bite is a quiet act of self-love.

Closing Reflection

"The first meal I enjoyed again after treatment wasn't fancy —
It was porridge with cinnamon and a smile." — Lina, 46

Nourishment is not about doing everything right.

It is about finding what feels gentle and supportive in this moment.

SMILOGIE TIP

Do not aim for perfect nutrition — aim for **kind nutrition.**

One comforting bowl of soup or one warm cup of Golden Milk is enough for today.

Gentle Prompt

What is one small way I can nourish myself today — through food, hydration, or a tiny ritual of care?

Affirmation

Food is comfort, connection, and care.
Each bite is a quiet act of self-love.

8
ENERGY & REST

"I honour my need for rest."

Smilogie Moment

There was a time I pushed through every dip in energy, believing rest meant weakness.

Life — and my body — taught me otherwise.

Rest is not failure; **it is medicine**.

So many women tell me they feel guilty for being tired.

But when we swap guilt for gentleness, rest becomes healing instead of shame.

A Gentle Note

Cancer treatment and hormonal changes can bring a deep, whole-body fatigue — the kind that sleep alone does not fix.

Energy may rise and fall unpredictably, and that can feel discouraging.

This tab helps you **work with your energy**, not against it.

When you pace your day, protect your energy, and allow rest without guilt, you begin to find a steadier rhythm — one that honours your healing.

Small restorations — a nap, a stretch, a soft smile — can renew you more than you expect.

Common Energy & Rest Wobbles

Wobble	Why It Happens	Gentle Supports
Cancer fatigue	Treatment effects, inflammation, low hormones	Pacing, planned rests, brief naps
Sleep disruption	Flushes, anxiety, medication timing	Evening rituals, cool room, screen-free wind-down
Energy crashes	Fluctuating stamina, blood-sugar dips	Balanced snacks, hydration, short walks
Rest guilt	"Should do more" thinking	Reframe: rest = recovery; schedule rests deliberately

Evidence Nugget

Cancer-related fatigue is one of the most common and treatable late effects; pacing and rest planning improve outcomes. (EONS 2022)

Pacing That Works

(so you avoid the boom-and-bust cycle)

The 4 Ps

- Prioritise → What truly matters today?
- Plan → Spread tasks gently through the day.
- Pace → Breaks before you crash.
- Posture → Sit or lie down for tasks when you can.

The 80% Rule

On good days, do **80%** of what you think you can.
Leave space for healing.

Traffic-Light Map

Choose tasks based on your current energy — not yesterday's.

🟢 **Green** (light energy)
Inbox triage • gentle stretch • fold laundry

🟡 **Yellow** (moderate)
Short walk • simple meal • tidy one area

🔴 **Red** (limited)

Appointments • errands • hosting • anything high-stimulation

Your colour can change during the day — switch guilt-free.

Sleep Sanctuary

- Consistent wake time — morning light resets your internal clock.
- 60–90 minute wind-down: dim lights, light reading, journaling.
- Bed = sleep/intimacy only. If awake >20 mins → move to a chair until sleepy.
- Ease caffeine after lunch.
- Avoid clock-watching.
- Night-flush soothers: light cotton, layers, cool room, fan, cool water by the bed.

Movement That Restores

Movement and rest are not opposites — they are partners.

- **Movement snacks** → 3–10 minutes, 2–4× daily (walk, stretch, yoga, tai chi).

- **Song Rule** → move for the length of one favourite song.

- **Breath-led movement** → inhale 4, exhale 6 to calm your system.

- **Start tiny** → consistency beats intensity.

Emerging research shows even two minutes of slow breathing or ankle pumps can lift circulation and reduce fatigue.

Quick Fuel for Steadier Energy

Pair **protein + fibre + healthy fat**:

- Apple + nut butter
- Yoghurt + berries + chia
- Hummus + carrots
- Roasted chickpeas / trail mix

  Small, balanced snacks = gentle, sustainable fuel.

Restorative Rituals

- Create a "rest corner" — blanket, scent, eye mask.
- 10-minute body scan or Yoga Nidra.
- Morning light if possible.
- Guilt-free nap: 10–20 minutes.
- Evening exhale: one page of "let it go" journaling.

One-Minute Reset

Smile softly →
4/6 breath × 4 →
Drop your shoulders →
Sip water →
Ask: Rest, snack, or stretch?
Choose the kindest one.

Energy & Rest Through the Smilogie Lens

S – Smile → Soften your shoulders and let your body know, "We're safe."

M – Mindfulness → Notice your energy colour before acting.

G – Gratitude → Thank your body for its signals, not just its stamina.

E – Energy → Protect it like a precious resource; plan rest first, then tasks.

Safety Check – Contact Your Team If...

- New or worsening breathlessness
- Chest pain or rapid heartbeat
- Significant swelling in legs or feet
- Fever, fainting, black/bloody stools
- Fatigue worsening despite rest

Ask about checks for

- Anaemia • Thyroid • B12 • Iron • Vitamin D • Medication side effects
- Sleep apnoea or restless legs (often overlooked)

Affirmation

I honour my need for rest.

SMILOGIE TIP

Rest is not wasted time — it is part of your strength.

Smilogie Reminder

Your energy is precious.
Protect it.
Pace it.
Honour it.

Reflection

Energy rises and falls like waves.

Listening — instead of resisting — helps your body guide you back to balance.

Gentle Prompt

Where could I allow myself a little more rest this week?

What small ritual could help me feel more restored?

9
REDISCOVERY BEYOND TREATMENT

"I am rediscovering myself, step by step."

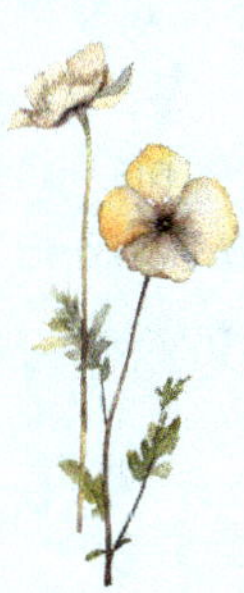

Smilogie Moment

A friend once said,

"Everyone expected me to celebrate when treatment ended — but I felt lost."

I have heard this many times, and felt it too.

When the storm passes, the quiet can feel heavier than the chaos.

Rediscovery is not about snapping back.

It is about slowly, gently meeting yourself again — without rush, pressure, or comparison.

A Gentle Note

Life after treatment is not about going back.

It is about discovering who you are now — with new strength, new softness, new needs, and new priorities.

This chapter makes space for that shift and reminds you:

Joy, confidence, identity, and connection are not lost.

They simply need to be nurtured in their new forms.

If you are unsure where to begin, survivorship nurses, counsellors, physiotherapists, and peer-support groups can guide you.

You do not have to figure this out alone.

"I am not who I was before — and that is okay.

There is something quietly powerful about beginning again."

Common Rediscovery Wobbles

Rediscovery Area	What It May Feel Like	Gentle Supports
Identity	"I don't feel like myself yet."	Journaling, values check-ins, reclaiming old joys, exploring new ones
Future	Fear of recurrence, "what now?"	Worry-window, If/Then plan, grounding, supportive community
Confidence	Body image, scars, fatigue	Body kindness, therapy, graded goals, peer support
Joy	Joy feels far away or muted	Tiny "Joy sparks," nature, music, quiet creativity

The Seasons of Rediscovery

You may move between seasons — gently, non-linearly.

Winter — cocooning, quiet, rest, protection
Spring — curiosity, small steps, lightness returning
Summer — energy, connection, exploration
Autumn — reflection, release, integration

> Each season has a purpose.
> None are wrong.

Survivorship — First Gentle Steps

Ask your team for a **survivorship or after-care plan** (a standard part of modern oncology care):

- Follow-up schedule & late-effects monitoring
- Bone, cardiovascular, thyroid, and vitamin checks
- Lymphoedema or physio referrals
- Menopause or hormone support
- Rehab or exercise guidance
- Dental & vaccination updates
- A clear list of who to call for what

These steps move you from **reactive care → proactive well-being**.

Evidence Nugget

Post-treatment adjustment is recognised as a major survivorship phase; graded re-engagement supports recovery.

— JCO Survivorship 2023

Fear of Recurrence (FoR) — A Kind Plan

1. Name it:

"This is a FoR moment."

2. Worry-window:

10 minutes → write → close the note.
Contain worry so the whole day isn't taken.

3. If/Then card:

If a new twinge appears → Then pause, breathe, and call your nurse if it lasts > 48–72 hours.

4. After scans:

Plan connection — a walk, coffee, call.
Do not sit alone with fear.

5. Evidence-based help:

Ask your team about:

- **ACT (Acceptance & Commitment Therapy)**
- **MBSR (Mindfulness-Based Stress Reduction)**
- **CBT for fear of recurrence**

These structured approaches teach emotional regulation, grounding, and self-compassion — cornerstones of survivorship well-being.

Rebuilding Body Trust

1. Sense

Where do I feel tight, tired, or okay?

2. Soothe

Breath, warmth/cool, stretch, rest.

3.Say

"Thank you, body. I'm listening."

Begin tiny: move for the length of one song.

Let comfort guide you: textures, scents, sounds that feel like "home."

> Relearning safety in your body is **neuro-retraining** — one of the most powerful forms of healing.

Return to Life & Work — At *Your* Pace

Start small
Return with hours you can repeat without crashing.
Plan rest first
Then layer tasks.

Micro-scripts

- "I can return for __ hours weekly; let's review in a month."
- "Afternoons are low energy for me — mornings are better."
- "I'll deliver A this week and B next week."

Social re-entry

- "I'll pop in for an hour."
- Leaving early is success, not failure.

Meaning, Joy & Purpose — Tiny but Real

- **Joy Sparks Journal** → one line a day: a laugh, a leaf, a kindness.

- **Breadcrumbs, not bucket lists** → one tiny new/old joy each week.

- **Mini service** → one message, one act, one kindness.

- **Creative calm** → doodle, knit, hum, plant seeds.

Evidence shows that small, consistent acts of joy and contribution reduce anxiety and lift well-being in survivorship.

Values Compass → Tiny Actions

Circle three values:
connection, play, steadiness, curiosity, compassion, courage

Then act within 48 hours:

- Connection → send a voice note
- Steadiness → sit in morning light for 3 minutes
- Play → dance while the kettle boils
- Courage → make one small plan for next week

Soft Goals That Stick (T I N Y)

Tiny • Invited • Near-term • Yes-able
Examples:

√ Walk to the end of the street

√ Text one friend

√ Water two plants

√ Read two pages

Small actions rebuild confidence in momentum.

Ritual — Closing the Treatment Chapter

Create your own ritual:

- Write a thank-you letter to your body
- Place hospital bracelets in a keepsake box
- Plant something new
- Light a candle and say,

"I carry the strength. I release the fear."

Rituals help your nervous system acknowledge that the chapter has turned.

Rediscovery Through the Smilogie Lens

S – Smile → Morning mirror: soft smile, "Welcome back, me."
M – Mindfulness → Three calm breaths before choices.
G – Gratitude → Note three "glimmers" each evening.
E – Energy → Plan rest first; protect your yes.

One-Minute Rediscovery Reset

Smile →
Inhale 4 / exhale 6 × 3 →
Name one value for the next hour →
Choose one tiny action: step outside, send a message, play a song.

Community & Connection

Rediscovery blooms in company: gentle exercise groups, expressive-arts sessions, coffee catch-ups, wellness circles.

Ask your oncology or survivorship centre about:

- peer-support groups
- community rehabilitation
- creative recovery programs
- psycho-oncology workshops

Connection is one of the strongest predictors of post-cancer resilience.

Sharing the path makes it lighter.

Closing Reflection

"My first real step forward wasn't a goal — it was a weekend walk."

"One morning, I smiled at my reflection and realised I was still here."

Rediscovery is not a finish line.

It is a rhythm — step by step, spark by spark, smile by smile.

Gentle Prompt

Which season of rediscovery am I in — winter, spring, summer, or autumn?

What is one spark of "me" I want to nurture this week?

Clinician Note — For Care Settings

Health professionals are welcome to share brief, unmodified excerpts of this guide in non-commercial patient-education settings, survivorship groups, or consultation rooms, provided attribution is included.

This chapter complements oncology, psycho-oncology, and integrative-care guidelines — offering accessible, compassionate practices rooted in evidence and human experience.

10
REFLECTIONS & SMILOGIE MOMENTS

"My smile is my quiet strength."

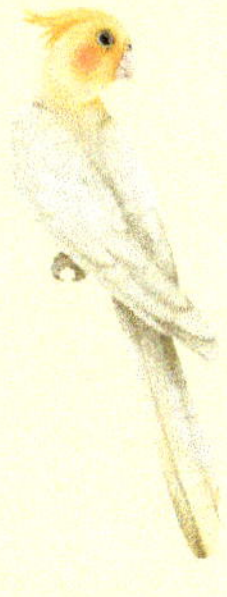

Smilogie Moment

When I began jotting down my wobbles and wins, I noticed something unexpected — I felt *lighter.*

Even a single line — a smile I spotted, a thought I wanted to keep — became a quiet sign of strength.

Over time, those tiny notes revealed a gentle truth:

I was moving forward, even on days it did not feel that way.

A Gentle Note

This final tab is yours — a small, calm corner to pause, soften, and gather what matters.

Writing helps feelings land.

It reduces overwhelm.

It helps the good moments shine through the noise.

Your Smilogie Touchstones are the tiny practices and phrases you can return to whenever you wobble.

Think of this section as a well — a quiet place to sip from when life feels dry.

How to Use This Tab (Your Way)

- **Daily** → one line, one spark, one smile.
- **Weekly** → a brief check-in using any prompt below.
- **Before/After appointments** → jot questions, feelings, or one thing that helped.
- **At bedtime** → a 3 • 2 • 1 journal or a soft closing reflection.

There is no wrong way — only *your* way.

Reflection Prompts

- What helped me feel more like myself this week?
- One small win I want to remember is...
- A shift I noticed in my energy, mood, or body...
- What does my heart need more of — and less of — right now?
- If I could whisper one kind word to myself today, it would be...

Smilogie 3•2•1 (60-Second Journal)

3 tiny gratitudes ("glimmers")
2 small wins (effort counts)
1 kindness I will offer myself tomorrow

Too tired?

One word each is enough.

Your nervous system responds to the *attempt*, not the perfection.

Wobble → Whisper (Reframing with Kindness)

Use these when your mind spirals:

"I'm not doing enough." →
"I am healing. Small steps are enough today."

"My body let me down." →
"My body is protecting me. I can listen gently."

"I should be over this." →
"Healing is not a line. I am allowed to be where I am."

Every whisper is a nervous-system reset.

Glimmers Log (Collect the Tiny Good)

Glimmers are small cues of safety — sunlight on your face, a kind text, soft sheets, a laugh.

List **three a day.**

Over time, your brain learns to spot them faster.

Clinically, this simple practice builds "neuroplastic gratitude" — rewiring the brain toward calm and safety.

Tiny Trackers (Data Without Pressure)

Mood → 😊 🙂 😕 ☹️

Energy → ● ● ● ●

Flushes → • • •

Water → □ □ □ □ □ □

Rest → □ nap □ wind-down □ in bed by . . . .

Circle, colour, tick — whatever feels easiest.

Tiny data → gentle awareness.

Smilogie Anchors (Tiny Practices for Wobbly Moments)

- **Pause & smile** — one soft breath, one soft smile.
- **5-Senses Grounding** — 1 see, 1 hear, 1 touch, 1 smell, 1 taste.
- **Gratitude Glimpse** — jot 3 tiny good things.
- **Compassion Check-In** — hand to heart: *"I am doing my best. That is enough."*
- **Energy Reset** — 2 minutes of slow breathing.

Each anchor signals safety to the body.

Self-Compassion Break (3 Lines)

1. **Notice** → "This is hard."
2. **Humanity** → "Others feel this too."
3. **Kindness** → "May I be gentle with myself right now."

Evidence-based: this sequence lowers cortisol and builds emotional resilience.

Build Your Affirmation Bank (That Feels 'True Enough')

Affirmations do not need to be perfect — just believable.
If a phrase feels too big, soften it:

"I love my body." →
"I am learning to care for my body."

"I'm fearless." →
"I can take this one step at a time."

The 51% Test
Does it feel at least slightly believable?
Then it counts.

Starter bank

- I am allowed to rest.
- Small steps count.
- I can meet today as I am.
- My smile is my quiet strength.

Monthly Pattern Finder

- **Highlights** → what helped most? What drained me?
- **Wins** → even tiny ones (asked for help, kept an appointment).
- **Next** → repeat one thing that worked.
Reflection turns patterns into wisdom.

SOS Card (for Heavy Days)

In 30–60 seconds:

1. Breathe (in 4, out 6) × 5
2. Sip water slowly
3. Text one safe person:

"I'm wobbly — can you sit with me by message?"

4. Step outside for 3 minutes of light or air
5. Circle one tiny next step:

- shower
- toast
- rest

If you ever feel unsafe or overwhelmed, contact your healthcare team or a trusted person immediately.

Smilogie Through Reflection

M – Mindfulness → writing helps you notice your inner world
G – Gratitude → collecting sparks builds resilience
E – Energy → reflection helps you place your precious energy where it matters

Reflection is not indulgence — it is recovery.

One-Minute Smile Scan

Smile softly →
Scan head to toe →
Choose one kindness (water / rest / move / message a friend) →
Do it now.
Tiny action → big nervous-system shift.

Closing Reflection

This companion began with a smile — and it ends with one too.
Every word you have read, and every line you write,
is part of your way back to yourself.

> *"Writing one line a night helped me see I was still healing — even on the quiet days."*

REFLECTIONS

"In this quiet space, I meet myself with kindness."

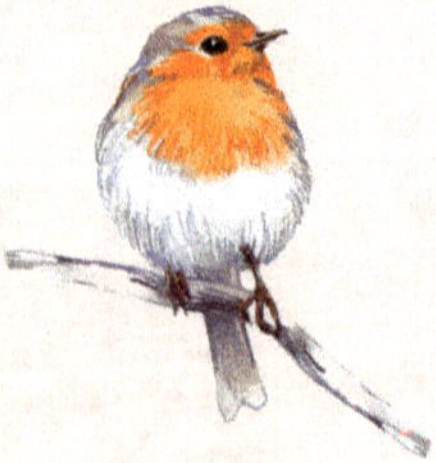

What helped me feel more like myself this week?

"Brushed my hair, wore real trousers, made it to noon before a nap — basically a comeback tour."

One small shift I am proud of is...

"One small smile. One small shift.
One substantial change."

A wobble I want to soften...

"Had a full-on cry over an advert. Then laughed. Emotional multitasking at its finest."

A moment of strength to remember...

....

....

....

....

....

....

....

....

....

....

....

....

....

....

....

....

....

....

"Rest is not weakness. It is wisdom."

What does my body need more of — and less of — right now?

"More naps, fewer 'I'm fine's."

If my heart could speak, it would ask for...

"Small sparks of joy light the way forward."

What brings me tiny sparks of joy?

"Fresh sheets, dark chocolate, saying no without apologising."

How will I remind myself I am more than my diagnosis?

"You're not starting over — you're continuing, with new strength and softness."

Little Tip

Reflection does not need to be perfect.
One line is enough.

Smilogie Reminder

Your pages are not for judgement —
They are a gentle mirror, reminding you of your strength.

Gentle Prompt

What is one Smilogie Touchstone I will carry into everyday life?

> *"At first I thought writing one line a night wouldn't help. But a week of tiny notes showed me I was moving forward after all."*

Clinician Note — Integration in Care Settings

Health professionals are welcome to use these journaling and reflection tools in group or 1:1 settings, provided attribution is included.

They align with evidence-based practices in self-monitoring, mindfulness, and self-compassion, shown to support mood, sleep, emotional regulation, and overall quality of life in cancer survivorship.

USEFUL RESOURCES

"The right support can lighten the load."

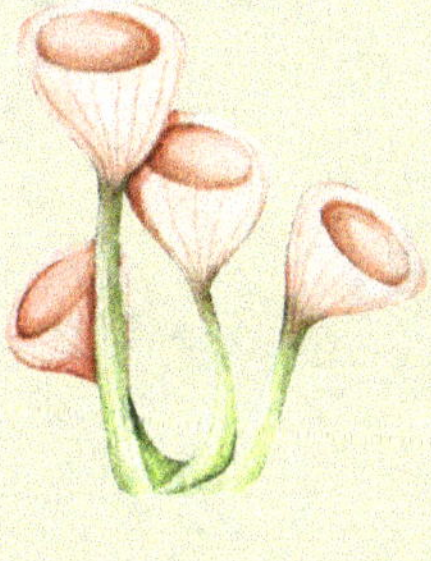

Smilogie Moment

I still remember the relief of finding the right person for a "silly" question.

Their kind, simple answer changed my whole week.

Often it is not *more* information we need but the **right information**, at the **right time**, from someone kind.

A Gentle Note

This tab is a small shortcut: trusted places to call, click, or visit when you want clarity, comfort, or your next step forward. Let your intuition lead.

Choose one or two that feel right today — that is enough.

**Evidence shows that timely signposting to reputable supports reduces anxiety and improves quality of life in cancer survivorship.*

* Mayer DK et al. CA Cancer J Clin (2021) 71: 246–275.

How to Use This Tab

(Without Overwhelm)

- **Star 3 go-tos:** one for medical info, one for emotional support, one for practical help.
- **Save one number** in your phone — your "first-call line."
- **Bookmark one directory** (therapist, physio, menopause specialist).
- **Accessibility nudge:** if energy is low, ask a friend to save links with you. Shared setup beats doing it alone.

Useful Resources (Start-Here Picks)

Medical & Cancer Information

- National cancer organisations (e.g., NCI, Cancer Research UK, American Cancer Society)
- Hospital cancer-centre patient libraries & oncology nurse helplines

Mind & Emotions

- Psycho-oncology services (ask your oncology team)
- National psychologist/counsellor directories
- Gentle guided-practice apps: Headspace, Calm, Insight Timer

Pelvic, Sexual & Intimacy Health

- Pelvic-health physiotherapists (women's-health/continence specialists)
- Cancer & intimacy hubs (dryness, pain, communication, body image)

Nutrition & Daily Living

- Evidence-based survivorship nutrition (WCRF/AICR & national orgs)
- Oncology-aware movement: gentle rehab, yoga, walking groups

Lymphoedema & Rehabilitation

- National lymphoedema associations & certified therapist finders
- Oncology rehab / physiotherapy directories

Menopause & Hormones (Oncology-Aware)

- Menopause charities & societies; national specialist finders
- Symptom-tracking apps (e.g., balance)

By Region

United Kingdom

- **Macmillan Cancer Support | Cancer Research UK**
- **NHS Talking Therapies** | BACP / UKCP therapist directories
- **The Menopause Charity** | British Menopause Society finder | balance app
- **Look Good Feel Better** workshops
- **Citizens Advice** for work, benefits, and treatment travel

United States

- **American Cancer Society | NCI Cancer Information Service**
- Psychology Today / APA therapist finders | hospital social-work teams
- **The Menopause Society (NAMS**) clinician finder
- Appearance-support programs (hospital or community)
- State cancer coalitions for transport & financial assistance

Ireland

- **Irish Cancer Society** (Freephone, Daffodil Centres, transport & welfare guidance)
- IACP / PSI / ICP therapist directories
- HSE menopause info | recognised specialist lists | **balance** app
- Look Good Feel Better Ireland
- HSE & **Citizens Information** for medical card, DPS, illness benefits

Books (Gentle, Grounded, Practical)

- *Mindfulness for Health* — V. Burch & D. Penman
- *After Cancer Treatment* — J. Silver, MD
- A brief CBT or ACT self-help guide you like (bring it to sessions)

  Examples only — choose what feels good for you.

Apps (Tiny Helpers in Your Pocket)

- **Calm / Headspace / Insight Timer** — breath, sleep, grounding
- **Balance** — menopause tracking + reports for appointments
- **Day One / Journey** — simple, soothing journaling

Websites (Evidence-Led)

- National cancer organisations (treatment, side-effects, survivorship)
- Menopause societies/charities (oncology-aware guidance on dryness, sleep, mood)
- Lymphoedema associations (self-care + therapist finders)
- Hospital cancer-centre patient pages (local services)

For other regions: search national cancer + menopause societies in your own language — many offer free helplines and survivorship resources.

Quick-Grab Page (Tear-Out or Screenshot)

My First Call

....

My Local Support Centre

....

My Directories

Therapist • Physio • Menopause specialist

....

My Calm App

....

Smilogie Lens for Resources

S – Start small → Choose one resource today.

M – Make it easy → Save a number / add a bookmark.

I – Invite support → Ask a friend to help if energy is low.

SMILOGIE TIP

You do not have to hold everything alone. One email, one call, one conversation can change the shape of a week.

Reminder

Support is not a luxury.
It is **part of your care**.

Plain-Language Note

These resources are for information, not for diagnosis or prescribing.

Always confirm personal care choices with your clinical team.

If You Are in Crisis

If you ever feel unsafe or overwhelmed, **call your local emergency number** or **hospital urgent-care line** immediately.

Closing Reflection

Which **one** resource will I explore this week to help myself feel more supported?

Clinician Note — Integration in Care Settings

Health professionals are welcome to share or reproduce this tab in patient-education sessions, provided attribution is included.

This section aligns with international survivorship-care guidelines and frameworks (EONS, Macmillan, ACS, ASCO), supporting:

- self-management
- informed decision-making
- emotional support
- safe navigation of care systems

These are recognised pillars of high-quality survivorship care.**

** ASCO / EONS Survivorship Framework (2022).

My Favourites Page

My go-to book

....

....

....

My go-to app

....

....

....

My go-to website

....

....

....

My first-call person / line

....

....

....

SMILOGIE TIP

Keep this page somewhere easy to reach. On heavy days, start with one familiar comfort from your list — often the simplest thing steadies the whole day.

A Note from Me to You

Thank you for opening this little book — and for trusting yourself enough to begin.

This was not a book of answers.

A tiny companion to remind you that **you are not alone**, and you are **stronger than you feel**.

Cancer and hormones bring wobbles, but you carry wisdom too.

Listen for your intuition — that quiet nudge that knows what feels right (and what does not).

Let it set your pace, and your next small step.

Your smile — soft, even shaky — is not a mask.

It is a sign whispering, "I'm still here."

No rush.

No perfection.

Just kindness toward your body, your mind, and your heart.

Trust your team.

And trust yourself.

If all you do today is breathe and drink a glass of water, that is enough.

With warmth,

Isy

A Tiny Intuition Check (Pocket Card)

Pause: one soft breath.
Ask: "What feels kind to me right now?"
Choose: one small step — rest / call / water / move / say no.
Notice: if your body softens, you are on your way.

Keep this card close — in your bag, journal, or phone notes. Intuition is not loud; it is **steady, kind, and wise**.

A Whisper Before You Go

"Cry, and the world cries with you.
Smile, and the world smiles too."

A smile is not pretending.
It is a small light—soft, sometimes shaky, always yours.

If it comes, let it rest beside you.
If it does not, let your breath be the gentle thing that stays.

For this moment, that is enough.

Stay Connected

- **Join** *The Smilogie Lift* on Facebook — a gentle community for shared stories and soft encouragement.
- **Explore more:** thesmilogiemethod.co
- **Follow:** @thesmilogiemethod

You are not alone.
We are in this together — one smile at a time.

Smilogie Side-Effects Spell

By one steady breath, shoulders drop.

By one warm sip, peace settles.

By one kind thought, the mirror softens.

By one gentle "no," room to breathe.

By one tiny step, strength returns.

By one small smile, courage lights up.

About the Author

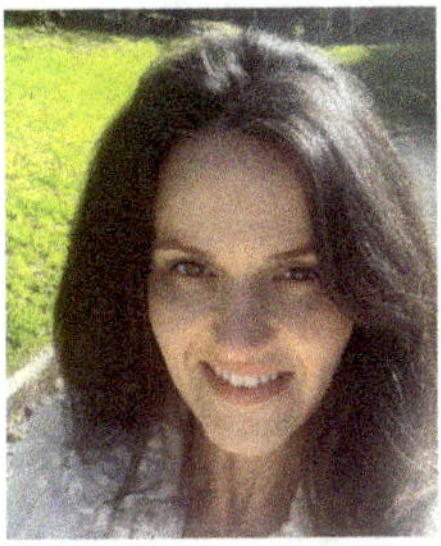

Isabelle (Isy) de Wouters d'Oplinter brings over thirty years of private coordination and a rich European heritage to her work. A certified Cancer Coach (Cancer Wellness Group) and a Health Coach graduate of the College of Naturopathic Medicine (UK), her approach is shaped by both evidence-based training and lived experience.

Smilogie began on a quiet morning when she caught her reflection and noticed a small, unexpected "I'm still here" smile.

It was not forced positivity — it was a moment of truth.

A reminder that even in the wobble, there is a spark of strength.

As she listened to women share their fears, fatigue, and flickers of hope, Isy longed to create support that felt lighter, simpler, and more human — something you could slip into a pocket when the world feels too heavy.

Not another overwhelming resource.

A companion.

Rooted in natural medicine, psycho-oncology coaching, and lived experience, the Smilogie Method blends micro-practices, emotional steadiness, and gentle community — offering women a way to feel calmer, clearer, and more connected to themselves.

Through her books, programs, and community, she offers a safe, steady place to feel seen, soothed, and gently guided back to what feels most alive — and toward the quiet trust of your own inner knowing.

My Favourites

(for you to fill in later)

Book I want to keep by my bed

....

....

....

App that helps

....

....

....

Website I trust

....

....

....

Local group / person I can call

....

....

....

These tiny anchors can become your personal support map — a reminder that help and hope are always within reach.

www.ingramcontent.com/pod-product-compliance
Lightning Source LLC
La Vergne TN
LVHW010319220926
848484LV00004BB/789
9781068249648